I0479797

# TERMINATING FEAR:
# A GUIDE TO OVERCOMING PHOBIAS AND FEARS

John K. Glover

# Table of Contents

# Chapter 1

## Describe Fear

One of the seven emotions that affect everyone on the planet is fear. When there is a genuine or imagined threat of harm—either physical, emotional, or psychological—fear develops. Although fear is typically regarded as a "bad" feeling, it plays a crucial part in keeping us safe since it prepares us to deal with impending danger.

## Being afraid

Three characteristics help to distinguish the frightening experience family:

Intensity: How serious is the danger that faces us?

When will the harm occur? Will it happen soon?

What steps, if any, may be made lessen or remove the threat?

Fear is reduced or eliminated when we can handle the situation. On the other hand, when we are unable to lessen the danger, this makes the terror worse. When a person is surprised, fear might occasionally follow right away. It frequently oscillates with fury.

What frightens us

The threat of injury, whether actual or imagined, is the primary cause of all forms of dread. Our physical, emotional, or psychological health may be at risk. While most of us have particular things that make us fearful, we can learn to be scared of almost anything.

Common causes of fear

obscurity - reduced visibility of the surroundings

flight and heights, interacting with others or being rejected, rodents, spiders, snakes, and other creatures

Dying and death.

Disorders and moods

If we experience consistent worry without understanding why it may be referred to as anxiety

rather than persistent terror. We are unable to remove ourselves or the real threat from the circumstance because we are unable to recognize the trigger.

Although anxiety is a common emotion for many people, it can be diagnosed as a disease when it is frequent, chronic, severe, and interferes with daily activities like work and sleep.

Read on for more information about phobias and anxiety.

Understanding fear.

Fear-related facial expressions

Fear frequently gets mistaken for a surprise when it manifests on the face.

While the eyebrows are lifted in both emotions, the eyebrows in a fear expression are straighter and more horizontal while the eyebrows in a surprise expression are raised and curled. In addition, fear lifts the upper eyelid higher than surprise, exposing more sclera (white of the eye). Last but not least, the lips are contracted and stretched in astonishment but more open and relaxed in fear.

Vocalizing one's fea

One's voice often has a higher pitch and a more strained tone when they are experiencing fear.

A person may also yell.

Feelings of dread

Shortness of breath and a feeling of chilly are frequent sensations. Additionally, it could cause shaking, sweating, and a tightening of the muscles in the arms and legs.

Pose of dread

The posture of dread might either be one of moving away or freezing—mobilizing or immobilizing.

The purpose of dread

The purpose of fear is always to prevent or lessen harm. We are capable of doing many things we wouldn't ordinarily be able to, or ready to do, halt the threat, depending on what we have learned in the past about what can protect us in dangerous situations.

Our attention is drawn to the current risk, which motivates us to take action to deal with it. In this sense, by compelling us to act without hesitation, terror might save our lives (e.g., jumping out of the way of a car coming at us).

Fear's predetermined evolutionary responses include fight, flight, and freeze.

## Responding to our fears

Despite being historically regarded as a "bad" emotion, fear plays a crucial part in keeping us safe. However, it might also keep us feeling confined and keep us from taking the actions we'd like to. While some people find dread almost intolerable and avoid it at all costs, others find enjoyment in terror and actively seek it out (i.e., watching a horror film).

## Addressing other people's fear

To appreciate, empathize with, and patiently reassure someone terrified of something we are not afraid of requires a highly developed capacity for compassion (most of us dismiss such fears). To acknowledge it and support them in coping, we do not have to share their fear.

## How Do We Physically Feel Fear?

Fear triggers physiological reactions in our bodies, just like many other fundamental emotions. Fear begins in the brain, and as it spreads throughout our bodies, we can modify and react to danger in the best way possible. Our bodies instinctively prepare us to either fight or run.

The amygdala, a region of the brain, is where fear first manifests. The amygdala stimulates areas involved in preparing for motor processes involved in fight or flight in response to threat stimuli, such as the sight of a predator, according to Smithsonian Magazine. Additionally, it causes the sympathetic nervous system and stress hormones to release.

We often go through three stages of the fear response because it is so automatic:

The evolutionary response that caused us to freeze was to remain hidden from a predator. If you're very terrified, you won't be able to halt your reflexive initial jump and stop your reaction to triggering stimuli.

Run: Our natural reaction is to flee from the source of our fear. You can move away from the trigger more rapidly thanks to adrenaline.

Fight: When you can't escape the source of your fear, you resort to violence. You benefit from adrenaline during this phase as well.

Of course, we no longer frequently need to hide from a predator, flee, or engage in combat when we sense fear. The physical reaction we feel is the same, though.

The majority of the physiological effects of fear are caused by modifications in our cardiovascular system.

Blood artery constriction and an increase in heart rate. Your breathing becomes faster, and your adrenaline level rises. Other organs, such as the liver and pancreas, may be impacted as a result of your body being forced into the fight-or-flight position.

Your muscles tighten because your body thinks you must be ready for a battle or flee. Even the ones at the bottom of your hair follicles, makes your hair stand on end. For this reason, prolonged fear and worry can cause persistent muscle discomfort.

Fear even triggers a biochemical reaction that has an impact on things like glucose levels and raises your risk of developing heart disease, kidney disease, eyesight issues, and other conditions. As a result, sustained physical stress from worry and dread can result in a variety of different physical symptoms and have an impact on your long-term health.

If your fear is intense, it may have negative impacts on your body. Although uncommon, it is possible to be deathly frightened. "Sudden, unexpected events can lead to a sharp rise in blood pressure and heart rate, putting those who already have cardiovascular disease in danger.

Fortunately, most fears are transient, but if you experience them frequently, it may be wise to take stock of your situation and seek support to move forward and prevent detrimental impacts on your health.

Understanding Your Fear And Getting Past It.

When prolonged or excessive, fear can paralyze you entirely and be bad for your health, but it also has many positive effects. For instance, terror might make you more conscious and help you think more clearly. This can be useful in conquering challenges in daily life if used properly. It's crucial to face your fear, overcome it, and use it to propel you forward.

Here are some strategies for utilizing your worry and fear to perform better in tense circumstances:

Accept your fear and use it to your advantage. Everybody experiences terrifying circumstances. Even if you don't react as you'd hoped in the heat of the moment, thinking back on what made the circumstance so difficult to handle can help you be more prepared to handle a similar situation in the future.

Realize that it may be advantageous. Fear can indicate that you're stepping outside of your comfort zone. You can persevere and gain strength by realizing that fear may be a sign that you are pushing yourself.

Grow to overcome obstacles. When you experience fear in your daily life, it may be a sign that you need to work on improving yourself. Consider how you might overcome the fears-inspiring challenges so that you are more equipped to do so.

Become proud. Fighting fear is challenging. It's an automatic process that could cause you to freeze and wear you out. If you persisted, think back on your bravery and be happy.

Phobias and fears.

When you're scared or extremely nervous, your body and mind move swiftly. These are some of the potential outcomes:

Your heart is beating quickly; it may feel erratic.

You exhale quickly.

Your muscles feel sluggish.

You perspire a lot

Your bowels feel loose or your stomach is churning.

It's challenging for you to focus on anything else.

You experience vertigo.

You experience a numb sensation.

You cannot eat.

You're sweating both hot and chilly.

Your mouth becomes dry.

Muscles become extremely tense. These events take place as a result of your body perceiving anxiety and preparing you for an emergency by increasing blood flow to the muscles, decreasing blood sugar levels, and enhancing your capacity to concentrate mentally. Over time, anxiety can cause some of the symptoms listed above as well as a more persistent feeling of fear. Additionally, anxiety can cause irritability, difficulty sleeping, headaches, difficulty focusing on work or making plans, issues with sex, and a loss of confidence.

Many things frighten us. Some fears can keep you safe. Fear of failure can motivate you to work hard so that you won't fail, but if the feeling is too powerful, it can also prevent you from working hard.

Each person is different in what they are scared of and how they react to it. Understanding your fears and their causes can be the first step toward resolving them.

Ten ways to overcome your worries

Here are 10 strategies to help you manage your regular fears and anxieties, no matter what it is that worries you.

These recommendations are for those who must manage regular concerns. See our page on generalized anxiety disorder if you have been given a diagnosis of an anxiety-related condition.

1. Take a break

Thinking is impossible when you're overcome by dread or anxiety. Take some time away so that you can physically calm down.

Take a 15-minute break from worrying by taking a walk around the block, brewing some tea, or taking a bath.

2. Continue breathing despite your fear.

The best course of action is to not fight it if your heartbeat quickens or your palms start to sweat.

Stay there and don't try to distract yourself; just feel the panic. The palm of your hand should be on your tummy as you take deep, calm breaths.

The intention is to remove the fear of fear by assisting the mind in becoming accustomed to handling panic.

Try this stress-reduction technique: breathing

3. Handle your phobias

Fears are only made scarier by being avoided. Whatever your fear, it should start to subside if you face it. For instance, it's best to enter a lift again the next day if you panicked the day before.

4. Think of the worst

Consider the worst-case scenario, which might be panicking and suffering a heart attack. then make an effort to imagine suffering a heart attack. It's simply not feasible. The more you pursue the fear, the faster it will flee.

5. Examine the proof.

Sometimes it is beneficial to confront fearful ideas. Ask yourself if you have ever heard of someone suffocating after becoming trapped in a lift, for instance, if you are afraid of doing so. Consider what you would say to a buddy who was experiencing a comparable phobia.

6. Don't strive for perfection.

Although life is stressful, many of us believe that our lives should be flawless. There will always be bad days and failures, and it's crucial to keep in mind that life is messy.

## 7. Think of a happy place.

Close your eyes for a moment and visualize a secure, tranquil environment. It might be a snapshot of you strolling along a lovely beach, curled up in bed with the cat next to you, or a pleasant childhood memory. Until you feel more at ease, let your good emotions calm you.

## 8. Discuss it

Sharing worries significantly reduces their terrifying power. If you are unable to speak with your partner, a friend, or a relative.

You could also attempt a telephone-based version of cognitive behavioral therapy.

## 9. Return to the beginning

Many people use alcohol or drugs as a self-medication for anxiety, but doing so will only make things worse. The best treatments for anxiety are frequently simple, everyday activities like a good night's sleep, a decent breakfast, and a walk.

10. Give to yourself.

Reward yourself at the end. Reinforce your achievement if you've already made the call you've been dreading, for instance, by rewarding yourself with a massage, a country walks, a meal out, a book, a DVD, or any other small gift that makes you smile.

Chapter 2

How can we make the most of our fear?

Fear can be a helpful feeling that serves to keep us safe from harm. It may inspire us to act and bring about the required adjustments in our life. Fear can assist us in focusing our attention and energy to more readily discover a solution when we are faced with a difficult circumstance. Additionally, fear might assist us in remembering crucial details and maintaining awareness in potentially hazardous situations. If we can learn to use our fear for good, it may be a potent instrument for propelling us toward our objectives.

The majority of us have experienced fear at some point or another. When you feel as though your current situation is in danger, you are threatened. The reflex is to run away or resist danger. We have had this tendency ever since our earliest days on earth. Fear can also be considered a motivator, as the force that compels us to act differently and cope with a challenging situation. The important thing is how we use fear: Whether we let it control us or decide to instead use its strength for good, igniting transformation in both ourselves and those around us!

I've learned through experience to confront my worries. What could go wrong, I tell myself at this time in my life. I say this because I've already experienced a lot of unpleasant things in my life, yet even if they were at times quite difficult, they didn't kill me. The truth is that if you don't confront your fear or a difficult scenario, a problem that might have had a very simple solution grows increasingly difficult.

Additionally, fear is a signal from your body that something needs to change. In the same way that pain alerts you to imminent trouble that probably has to be handled, it is your body's reaction to an unpleasant circumstance. Fear is an essential survival strategy. Consider fear as the sixth sense. Fear alerts you to the possibility of something horrible happening. Fear is warning you to shift course and pivot, or to start preparing yourself for a particularly trying circumstance.

Since wonderful things rarely come easily, fear helps prepare your body both emotionally and physically for better opportunities in life. Because it is our body's method of alerting us that we might need to modify something, fear can be a good thing. Fear is ultimately just a feeling, and not all emotions are negative. Fear encourages you to take on more in life, which results in a deeper experience.

Fear can be incapacitating. We can get paralyzed by our fear of failure, rejection, or just uncertainty. When we become prisoners of our thoughts, we could find ourselves in a frustrating and unfulfilling corner. On the other side, there is a benefit to dread. Fear prevents us from acting dangerously, such as walking off the top of a 16-story building, from a survival perspective. Thank you, height phobia. The fear of not accomplishing goals or falling short of a vision can motivate us if we focus our efforts in the appropriate direction.

Here are some facts about fear that will help you manage it rather than letting it rule your life.

1. Acknowledge that most of your anxieties are unfounded

Sometimes our thoughts wander and project. We are incredibly capable of speculating, imagining, and marveling. Given that creativity is the source of invention, this may be a plus. When the scenarios we envisage cause fear, it can also become problematic. Worst-case scenarios are easy to envision. The "what if" aspect tends to paralyze us into inaction.

Some minds seem to dwell more than others in the murkier side of "what if." You eventually just have to accept that the things you're worrying about are improbable and go on. Analyzing the concerns you've had in the past that didn't come true can help you get over your current ones rather than giving in to the dread in your head. When you realize that your fear is unfounded, the barrier is broken and you can move forward.

2. Recognize that even your sensible anxieties are probably unfounded.

Even if our anxieties are justified and grounded in truth, much of life is a mental conflict rather than a physical one. Even the majority of the plausible possibilities we conjure up will never materialize. True enough, not even close.

Let's remember that the possibilities for the future are only that for those of us who manage to frighten ourselves with them. You won't experience the vast majority of embarrassment, disgrace, terrible diseases, or horrific ways to pass away. Life's tragedies are frequently unforeseeable and inescapable. Stop letting it ruin your life, then!

You'll feel more at ease once you accept this, and it might even inspire you to do new things. You're free to live life more vibrantly without the sense of impending catastrophe.

3. Recognize that sometimes you will experience actual fear, but you will overcome it.

Even the greatest, most cautious, and healthiest among us experience bad things. But even if we do experience fear, it's probably not as awful as we initially believed. The guy you were seeing was still seeing his ex-girlfriend, you utterly failed an interview, or you're a lousy executive assistant. Even though these situations can be unpleasant at the time, everything up to and including death is not the end of the world.

You can do it. You will succeed. Additionally, many nightmares that come true eventually lose their impact. Typically, it's never as bad as you anticipated, and even when it is, it usually improves. Even in the face of extremely horrible occurrences, you'll surprise yourself with your sincerity.

4. Recognize that facing your concerns might help you grow

These occasionally unpleasant experiences also aid us in defining what we don't want. It's possible that you don't fit the office's vibe, the weepy artist wasn't what you thought he would be, or being someone's nanny isn't in your destiny. Even worse things exist.

Use these encounters as a way to reflect and declare, "This didn't work. It didn't fit, that. What else is there, then? We have adapted beings. You have this strength within you that comes from nature; embrace it, and you will conquer even your darkest worries.

5. Recognize that you'll succeed at the tasks you're putting off out of fear.

There is occasionally a learning curve. Don't be alarmed by it. In fact, it's fantastic if you feel terrified because you're being challenged or attempting something new! Growing pains are a byproduct of development.

The reality is that the lessons you've already acquired in life reinforce one another and help you become more proficient at new tasks. And you can take in a lot of fresh information. There isn't much you can't learn, and in all honesty, you probably already do it well. Your only regret will be that you didn't get started sooner. A little soreness and tension are temporary. But catching up on time? That is quite difficult. Do it now. You'll be alright.

6. Attempt to channel your anxiety over not being "good enough" and use it as motivation to work more.

The initial action in whatever you invest time and energy in is the most difficult. After a mile of a daily walk, you get into a rhythm and stop worrying about how difficult it was to begin; you are just focused on doing the task at hand.

It might be intimidating to try something new, whether it's learning a new computer program or increasing one's physical fitness or health. Negative self-talk or the nagging doubt in the back of your mind that you won't succeed can prevent you from ever attempting. But in actuality, failing to try will not haunt you as much as failing to try at all.

When you begin to doubt your abilities, gather that anxiety and use it to motivate yourself to achieve your objectives. Instead of allowing yourself to give in to the sensation of anxiety growing over your chest, deliberately acknowledge that once you start, the majority of your difficulty will quickly be reduced to something manageable. Don't accept failure or complacency; instead, utilize your fear of them to overcome them. Use the dread that someone else is achieving your dreams to keep your attention on your own.

We have been taught that envy and jealousy are negative emotions, and to some extent, this is true. You waste time whenever your attention is diverted from living your own life to someone else's. Unless you can channel those emotions into concentration.

Do you observe others leading the life you desire? Jealous? Never be! Recognize that they have many of the same human weaknesses, insecurities, and flaws as you. Instead of giggling with envy over something you want for yourself, consider why you are feeling this way. You will be able to focus on issues like "What measures can I take to make these things a reality in my own life?" if the response is, "I want to travel, be in a great relationship, or establish my own business."

You'll discover that once you focus your efforts on achieving your objectives, you won't have time to be jealous of other people's successes. When you do learn what your classmates are doing, you'll be delighted for them since you won't be constrained by your shame or inferiority complex.

8. Keep in mind that failures are inevitable, but that failure is the best teacher. You will err from time to time. It's normal to fail throughout the process. Any successful person will admit that they have failed at least once.

These failure stories are frequently coupled with later amazing accomplishments. The failure provided some profound insight or fixed a poor strategy for solving an issue. Receiving a resounding "no" from the people in our lives, the market, or the universe is the only test of whether something works and is a teacher as potent as the sting of failure.

9. Give yourself a high five.

Congratulate yourself for having the courage to overcome your anxiety and acknowledge the strength it takes to do so. And use that knowledge to your advantage in the future to be stronger. Consider the things you formerly feared and how you conquered them in the past. Examine how you were correct about the things you knew you were meant to do and how you were incorrect about some things that used to paralyze you. Your accomplishments will steadily surpass your insecurities, and you'll find that new fears become less scary.

Chapter 3

Knowledge of the Science of Fear

Fear is a common thread that flows through every one of our lives, whether it is dread of success, rejection, or just fear that we are not enough. If we allow it, fear can keep us imprisoned in the familiar and predictable, preventing us from realizing our full potential. Living in fear creates a catch-22 situation where you are unhappy with the current quo but hesitant to seek out something better.

However, there is another way that fear can be put to good use, enabling us to overcome our irritation and live the life we want. Yes, if you let it, fear may be used as a tool to achieve fulfillment. Learn how to avoid living in dread or, even better, how to turn fear into your greatest source of inspiration.

TYPES OF TERROR

You need to be aware of the psychology of fear to actively combat it and cease living in it. Fear and anxiety do have a place in a normal human psyche, up to a degree. A normal feeling, acute fear alerts you to a possible danger to your physical or emotional security. If you've ever been in an accident, felt like you were being followed, or encountered another urgent hazard, you've probably noticed that your heart begins to beat more quickly. Your veins start to pump with adrenaline. You are more alert than usual, which enables you to act quickly to save yourself or other people. A natural reaction that assisted our ancestors in surviving was acute dread.

When the acute fear reaction turns hypersensitive, another kind of terror develops. Chronic fear, also known as indirect fear, develops when we are repeatedly exposed to unpleasant but low-intensity experiences. We could consume a lot of news about conflict, political strife, or the most recent medical discoveries, leading us to unjustifiably anticipate unfavorable outcomes. Contrary to acute terror, persistent fear can inhibit our body's natural response to save us, leading us to feel as though an outside force is needed to "save" us.

WHY DO I RUN AWAY FROM FEAR?

Harvard University research indicates that in the previous 12 months, little over 19% of the population had an anxiety problem. They rank among the most prevalent psychological conditions in the US. Our deep-seated anxiety problems in the modern world are often brought on by continuous fear, for which everything from the media to caffeine has been held responsible. But dwelling in a place of blame has never made anyone's troubles go away. It's time to take control of your feelings and make changes in your life.

What is the most effective technique to manage fear, then? You have to learn how to move with it. Tony explains in the video below how to control your fear rather than letting it control you.

Symptoms of living in fear

Would you believe that a large number of people live their lives unaware that they are experiencing fear? Because comfort and terror are frequently mistaken, we start to feel at ease in our lives and believe that we are content and happy. One of the Six Human Needs is a certainty, but when we get too comfortable with it, it tends to hold us back. Here are a few indicators that you are experiencing fear:

Our survival instinct is fear. Some people (horror movie buffs and fans of roller coasters) love it while others stay away from it. Ever ponder the reasons why?

Concern Is Physical

Although fear is felt in the head, it also causes a powerful physical response in the body. Your brain's amygdala, a little structure in the center, begins to function as soon as you perceive fear. Your neurological system becomes alert, which activates the terror reaction in your body. Cortisol and adrenaline, two stress hormones, are released. Your heart rate and blood pressure rise. Your respiration quickens. Blood flows out from your heart and into your extremities, altering even your blood flow, which makes it simpler for you to start punching people or running for your life. Your body is getting ready to either fight or run.

Fear might cloud your judgment.

Some of your brain's processes are accelerating, while others are slowing down. It becomes challenging to think clearly or make sound decisions when the cerebral cortex, the part of the brain that controls reasoning and judgment, detects fear. As a result, you can panic and scream when an actor in a haunted home approaches you since you can't make yourself understand that the danger is imaginary.

Fear Can Become Enjoyment

But why do fans of roller coasters, haunted houses, and horror films like to get sucked into those tense, frightening situations? Considering that the thrill doesn't always cease when the ride or movie does. Your body and brain continue to be stimulated thanks to the excitation transfer process even after your frightful experience has ended.

Your brain will create more dopamine, a neurotransmitter that induces pleasure after a contrived fear encounter.

Phobia Is Not Fear

After viewing "Jaws," if you feel a little nervous about swimming in the water, the film succeeded in its goal. However, if the mere concept of lounging on the beach leaves you feeling scared, traumatized, and unable to function, you might be going through more than just fear.

It's easy to tell the difference between fear and phobia. Fears are frequent responses to situations or things. However, fear turns into a phobia when it impairs your capacity to carry out daily tasks and keep up a stable standard of living. You may have a phobia if you start going out of your way to avoid things like water, spiders, or people.

Fear Protects You

We all experience fear naturally and biologically, and we must do so because it keeps us safe.

Humans see fear as a complicated emotion that has both positive and negative effects. Speak with your primary care provider if a fear or phobia interferes with your life in a bad or uncomfortable way. They can help you determine the type of treatment you may require.

My fear dissuades me from taking a chance. I don't take action when I'm terrified. I'm in defense mode. I become stuck.

I think my finest days are behind me because of my fear. I feel irrelevant and washed up after being overcome by fear.

I can continue to be toxic and unhealthy because of my fear. Because I'm immobile and stuck, I'm constantly exposed to unhealthy situations. even if I hope for improvement. There is no change. I'm not altering my behavior in any way.

Fear undermines the potential of hope and draws my attention to my skepticism. Instead of paying attention to the possibility that my circumstances may change, I concentrate and spend time on what it is I am terrified of. Most likely, they will evolve.

Fear diminishes my sense of worth. I start looking for explanations as to why my circumstances are as they are. I fail to recognize my worth. It turns into a vicious circle.

Fear makes me apathetic, depressed, and lonely. I become caught up in a vicious cycle of shame. Instead of being vulnerable and confiding in my friends and community, I find reasons to justify why things are as bad as they are.

Fear steadily robs me of my life and pleasure. I find that when I become more and more worn out, I just want to be alone myself. Depression begins to take hold.

I continue to support my circumstances out of fear. I go from change mode to survival mode. Instead of adopting a courageous mindset, I adopt an enduring attitude.

I believe that this is the best I can do because of fear. I am deceived into thinking that I have passed my prime.

I'm held captive by fear till things grow even worse. I conduct myself as though there are no options. I've bought into the falsehoods that have been going through my thoughts.

Perfectionism. We hide behind the need to be perfect to prevent ourselves from experiencing real closeness and connection. It is also the lowest standard in the world, as Tony stated, due to its impossibility.

Settling. On the other side, settling for less than you deserve is a strong sign that your need for certainty is taking control of your life. You're living in dread if you don't have a remarkable, passionate relationship and a job you adore.

Procrastination. Delaying tasks perpetually till "tomorrow" or "when I have more time" is a common strategy for those who live in fear. Stop coming up with justifications and start working toward your goals.

becoming numb. Living in a beautiful state makes it unnecessary to use drugs or drink to have fun. You have an open mind, control your emotions, and experience unadulterated delight every day.

How to stop fearing anything

When you have a persistent fear, you don't just feel anxious; you live it. The fear response develops into an unhealthy way of life that affects everything you think, feel, and do. Fear keeps you mired in a vicious cycle of failure and frustration. The good thing about fear is that it usually comes with unpleasant emotions that make you want to avoid it.

Don't allow fear to rule your actions. There are various ways to quit living in dread, including exercising, taking care of oneself, and getting professional assistance. You can find ways to overcome your anxieties and find serenity when you commit to addressing them.

The truth is that I haven't been paying attention to the actual truth. I've been concentrating on my worry and fear. All of us go through a range of emotions each week. Some of us are engaging in mental patterns that are incredibly harmful to us. Every time we experience fear, we must confront it head-on with the truth. Keep in mind that everyone has a pre-programmed operating system for fear. Fear arises from the way we interpret our experiences and think about them. Our thoughts are on the wrong things when we are caught in a loop of unhealthy and false beliefs. What is reality? frantically look for the truth.

1. Why is fear such a potent emotion?

Fear is a primal, strong, and common human emotion. It involves a widespread biological reaction as well as a strong individual emotional reaction, according to psychological study. Whether the threat is psychological or physical, fear serves as a warning when danger is present.

Worry can come from both genuine and imagined hazards. Real threats can sometimes be the source of fear. While in some circumstances fear is a natural reaction when it is excessive or out of proportion to the threat, it can also cause anguish and disturbance.

Some mental health illnesses, such as panic disorder, social anxiety disorder, phobias, and post-traumatic stress disorder, can also show symptoms of fear (PTSD).

Biochemical and emotional responses to a perceived threat make up the two main components of fear.

Reaction in Biochemistry

Fear is a healthy feeling and a form of survival. When we encounter a threat, our bodies react in particular ways. Fear causes us to physically react by perspiring, speeding up our hearts, and becoming more alert due to high adrenaline levels.

Your body prepares for either fighting or flight with this physiological reaction, which is often referred to as the "fight or flight" response. This metabolic process is probably a result of evolution. It is a natural reaction that is essential to our survival.

An emotional reaction

On the other hand, each person's reaction to fear is very unique. Feeling fear in certain conditions, such as when you watch scary movies, can be perceived as fun because it triggers some of the same chemical reactions in our brains as good emotions like happiness and enthusiasm do. 2

Some people live for extreme sports and other thrill-seeking circumstances that make them anxious. Some people react negatively to the emotion of fear and avoid frightening situations at all costs.

Although the bodily response is the same, depending on the individual, the experience of terror may be interpreted positively or negatively.

Signs of Fear

Fear frequently causes both physical and emotional side effects. While everyone experiences fear differently, the following are some typical indicators and symptoms:

chest pain

Chills

mouth ache

Nausea

a quick heartbeat

breathing difficulty

Sweating\sTrembling

uneasy stomach

People may suffer psychological symptoms such as feeling overwhelmed, disturbed, out of control, or a sensation of imminent death in addition to the physical signs and symptoms of terror.

Identifying Fear

If your feelings of fear are extreme and persistent, speak with your doctor. To make sure that your worry and fear are not caused by an underlying medical problem, your doctor may undertake a physical examination and blood testing.

Your doctor will also inquire about your symptoms, including their duration, severity, and circumstances that often bring them on. Your doctor may determine that you have an anxiety disorder such as a phobia based on your symptoms.

Phobias A tendency to develop a fear of fear might be one part of anxiety disorders.

3 Those who suffer from anxiety disorders may become worried that they will feel terror, but most people typically only feel fear when it is associated with a scary or dangerous circumstance. They actively try to avoid their fear reactions because they see them as negative.

An abnormal fear response is called a phobia. The thing or circumstance that is causing the dread is not dangerous. Even though you are aware that the worry is unwarranted, you are powerless to stop yourself. As the fear of terror reaction sets in, the fear tends to get worse with time.

Fear and Phobia: How They Differ Reactions to Fear Causes of Fear

There is no single, fundamental basis for fear since it is so multifaceted.

4 Some phobias may be the outcome of trauma or traumatic experiences, while others may be the result of dread of something completely different, like losing control. Other phobias, such as a fear of heights because they make you feel lightheaded and queasy, may arise as a result of physical symptoms.

Common things that make people dread include:

specific things or circumstances (spiders, snakes, heights, flying, etc)

Future activities

Imaginary things

Actual environmental risks

Not knowing

Due to their role in survival, some anxieties are often natural and may have evolved. Others are acquired and linked to associations or upsetting events.

Different Fears

Fear is a characteristic of several distinct forms of anxiety disorders, such as:

Agoraphobia

Disorder of generalized anxiety

panic attack

trauma-related stress disorder (PTSD)

Disorder of separation anxiety

Disordered social anxiety

Particular phobia

List of Phobias and Fear Management

Familiarity, which results from repeated exposure to identical circumstances, can significantly lessen the terror response. Some phobia treatments use this strategy as their foundation since it works to gradually reduce the fear reaction by making it feel familiar.

Treatments for phobias that are based on the psychology of fear frequently include methods like flooding and systematic desensitization. Both methods diminish fear by influencing your body's physiological and psychological reactions.

Continually Desensitizing

To undergo a series of exposure situations gradually is known as systematic desensitization. For instance, if you're afraid of snakes, your therapist and you might spend the first session discussing snakes.

Your therapist would guide you gradually throughout subsequent sessions as you practiced handling a live snake, playing with toy snakes, and looking at pictures of snakes. This is typically done in conjunction with learning and using fresh coping mechanisms to control the fear response.

Flooding

This kind of exposure technique has the potential to be very effective.

Flooding because you must unlearn your phobia because it is a taught behavior.

In a safe, controlled atmosphere, you are exposed to a great deal of the dreaded objects or circumstances when you flood, and this exposure lasts for a long time until the fear passes. For instance, even if you're frightened of flying, you'd still board a plane.

The goal is to push you through your severe anxiety and possibly panic to a point where you must face your fear and ultimately come to terms with the fact that you are fine. This can aid in fusing a dreaded event—flying on a plane—with a positive response—you're not in danger—to help you overcome your fear.

Even if these treatments have a great chance of success, it's crucial that such confrontational methods only be used under the supervision of a qualified mental health expert.

Managing Fear

You can also take actions to assist you to deal with fear in daily life. These methods concentrate on controlling the negative behavioral, emotional, and bodily impacts of fear. Among the things you can accomplish are:

Obtain social assistance. You can better control your feelings of dread by surrounding yourself with encouraging people.

Engage in mindfulness. Even if you can't always control your emotions, mindfulness can help you control them and replace unhelpful thoughts with constructive ones.

Use stress-reduction methods including progressive muscle relaxation, visualization, and deep breathing.

Fear is a healthy human emotion that can help you avoid danger and get ready to act, but it can also cause feelings of anxiety that endure for a longer period. Discovering techniques for managing your fear can make it easier for you to deal with these emotions and keep anxiety from taking hold.